Biomimetics in Maxillofacial Surgery

CV CONTENT VIBES
PUBLISHERS • PRINTERS • AGGREGATORS

About the Authors

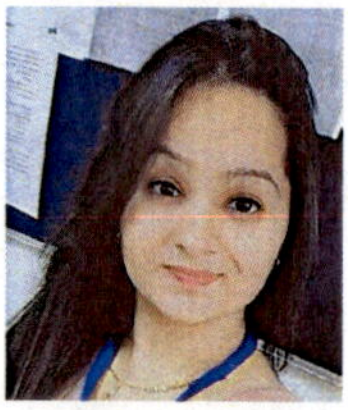

Dr. Aditi Rapriya is currently pursuing post-graduation in the field of Oral and Maxillofacial Surgery at SGT Medical College, Hospital and Research Institute, Gurugram, Haryana. She has completed her graduation from Pt B.D. Sharma University of Health Sciences, Rohtak in 2018. Armed with an insatiable curiosity and a dedication to advancing surgical techniques, she has a keen interest in the field of Facial Trauma, Head and Neck Oncology, Facial Aesthetics, Orthognathic Surgeries, Microvascular Surgeries and reconstruction. She is dedicated to her field exemplified by her status as a student life member of the AOMSI.

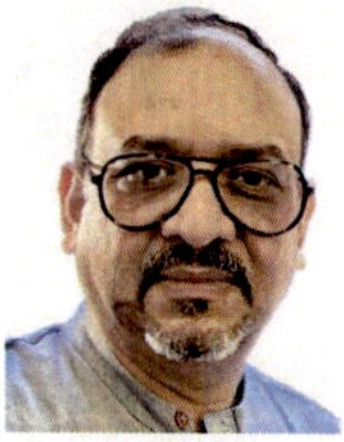

Dr. Sanjeev Kumar has an experience of 32 years in the field of Oral and Maxillofacial Surgery. An alumnus of Dr. R. Ahmed Dental College at Kolkata, Dr. Sanjeev completed his M.D.S. from Govt Dental College at Ahmedabad in 1991. He further refined his skills at U.K, where the Royal College of Surgeons and Physicians, Glasgow awarded him the FDSRCPS. He has also been awarded the Fellowship of Indian Board of Oral & Maxillofacial Surgery in 2008. Currently, Dr. Sanjeev is heading the Department of Oral & Maxillofacial surgery at FDSC, SGT University. The department caters to the training requirements of BDS, MDS and PhD students under his guidance. He is an accredited surgeon with the Smile Train organization and is associated with the Nav Muskaan project at SGT University which treats children with cleft lip and palate free of cost. He was the founder President of Delhi Chapter of Oral and Maxillofacial Surgeons of India. Dr. Sanjeev is a life member of AOMSI since past 14 years and is involved actively in their fellowship program and IBOMS examination. He is also a National faculty for AOCMF, the flagship International body involved in training surgeons in osteosynthesis techniques. He regularly conducts courses for AOCMF in various locations in India

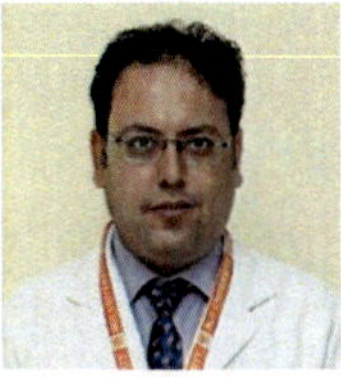

Dr. Varun Arya did BDS as well as MDS from SGT Dental College Hospital and Research Institute, Gurugram, Haryana. He has 36 publications in national and international journals. He has presented scientific papers at International level and poster at national level and is a member of various associations. Interests into a wide Facial and Aesthetics Medicine for Oral and Maxillofacial Surgeon, and spectrum of cases ranging from minor surgical procedures, oral implants, pathologies, major surgical procedures like trauma, TMJ cases, cleft lip and palate cases, orthognathic surgery, maxillofacial reconstruction and carcinoma and rhinoplasty procedures.

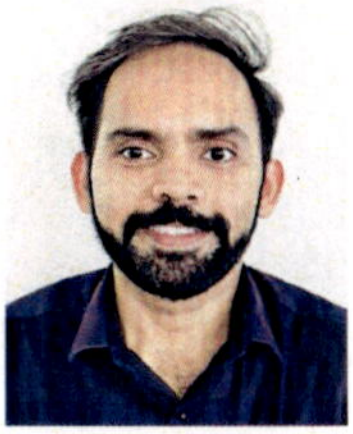

Dr. Ajay Das T. has done his BDS from Sree Mookambika Institute of Dental Sciences, TamilNadu in 2006 and went on to pursue MDS in Oral and Maxillofacial Surgery from Annamalai University from 2012. He has completed Fellowship in Dental Implants from ICOI, USA and also is a Fellow of Indian Board of Oral and Maxillofacial Surgery. He has academic experience of 9 years and is currently working as an Associate Professor at SGT University, Gurugram. He has keen interest in Maxillofacial Trauma, Orthognathic Surgery, Dental Implants, TMJ pathologies etc.

Biomimetics in Maxillofacial Surgery

Advancing Maxillofacial Surgery through Biomimetics

Aditi Rapriya
Sanjeev Kumar
Varun Arya
Ajay Das T.

CV CONTENT VIBES
PUBLISHERS • PRINTERS • AGGREGATORS

CONTENT VIBES
PUBLISHERS • PRINTERS • AGGREGATORS

1168, Sector 13, Urban Estate
Karnal-132 001, Haryana
Tel: 91-84470 75807, 18440 41168
Email: contentvibesppa@gmail.com
www.contentvibes.in

Print ISBN: 978-81-97781-59-9

ebook-ISBN: 978-81-97781-52-0

Preface

The preface of this book offers an in-depth look into the realm of implantable biomaterials for craniofacial reconstruction, highlighting several critical aspects:

1. Unique Challenges in the Craniofacial Region

- **Dynamic Mechanical Stresses**: Craniofacial muscles exert varied and dynamic mechanical forces, creating a unique challenge for implantable biomaterials.
- **Aging Effects**: Aging leads to a loss of skin elasticity and tissue sagging, which further complicates reconstruction efforts.

2. Traditionally Used Methods

- Autogenous Bone Grafts: Historically, autogenous bone grafts have been the go-to method. However, they come with significant drawbacks:
  - Harvesting difficulties
  - Time consumption
  - Donor site morbidity
  - Potential for bone resorption

3. Advancements in Alloplastic Materials

- Improved Biocompatibility: Recent advancements have led to the increased adoption of alloplastic bone substitutes, which are materials made from synthetic substances.
- Combined Use: These materials are often used alongside autologous (from the patient), allograft (from a donor), or other synthetic materials to enhance surgical outcomes.

4. Proactive Design of Biomaterials

- Targeted Responses: Current trends emphasize designing biomaterials that elicit specific, desirable responses from tissues and cells.
- Goals:
  - Faster healing
  - Reduced rejection rates
  - Enhanced biocompatibility

5. Future Directions and Challenges

- Long-term Performance: There is a need to improve the long-term performance and biocompatibility of these materials.
- Infection Control: Addressing infection control remains a significant challenge.
- Mechanical Properties: Optimizing the mechanical properties of biomaterials to withstand craniofacial muscle forces is essential.
- Integration with Living Tissues: Developing materials that integrate seamlessly with living tissues is a primary focus.
- Innovative Formulations: Future research aims to develop innovative biomaterial formulations and explore new applications in tissue engineering.

6. Overall Evolution of the Field

- Rapid Advancement: The field is rapidly evolving, driven by clinical needs and technological advancements.
- Shift Towards Alloplastic Substitutes: There is a notable shift towards using alloplastic substitutes to overcome the limitations of autogenous bone grafts and improve material biocompatibility.
- Interdisciplinary Collaboration: Progress in craniofacial surgery relies heavily on interdisciplinary collaboration between materials science, biology, and clinical medicine.

Summary

The preface provides a comprehensive overview of the current state, challenges, and future directions in the field of craniofacial biomaterials. It emphasizes the importance of innovation and collaboration in advancing surgical outcomes in this specialized field.

Acknowledgment

ॐ कृष्णाय वासुदेवाय हरये परमात्मने॥
प्रणत: क्लेशनाशाय गोविंदाय नमो नम:॥

"No one who achieves success does so without the help of others. The wise and confident acknowledge this help with gratitude."
–Alfred North Whitehead

Though words are seldom sufficient to express gratitude and feelings, it gives me an opportunity to acknowledge those who helped me during my post-graduation days.

First, I bow with reverence to thank God who enriched me with such a golden opportunity and infused the power in my mind to fulfill the task assigned to me.

Firstly, I express my sincere and deepest gratitude to the Professor and Head of the Department

Dr. Sanjeev Kumar who ploughed through several preliminary versions of my text, making critical suggestions, and posing challenging questions. His expertise, invaluable guidance, constant encouragement, affectionate attitude, understanding, patience, and healthy criticism added considerably to my experience. Without his continual inspiration, it would have not been possible to complete this library dissertation.

I take this opportunity to express my deep sense of gratitude and respectful regard to my guide

Dr. Varun Arya and co-guide **Dr. Ajay Das T,** for guiding me through this topic of the dissertation and for their meticulous supervision, valuable guidance, encouragement, and critical appreciation. Their consistent guidance has helped me pave the way to various fruitful opportunities.

I sincerely acknowledge my gratitude towards my eminent teachers who have been a wonderful guiding torch in all my endeavours and a tremendous source of inspiration and constant navigation with their gentle guidance **Dr. Alok Bhatnagar, Dr. Jitender Kumar, Dr. Sunil Gulia, Dr. Minerva Singh, Dr. Manu Gupta, and Dr. Monika Tanwar.**

I want to express my thanks for the persistent help and support from my batchmates **Dr. Isha, Dr. Prabodh, Dr. Divanshi, Dr. Geetu** and **Dr. Partishtha.** I would also like to thank my juniors **Dr. Alaida, Dr. Sameera, Dr. Virender, Dr. Angel, Dr. Habiba** and **Dr. Zenab** and super juniors **Dr. Deepak. Dr. Bobby, Dr. Kajol, Dr. Neelakshi, Dr. Swati** and **Dr. Supayan** for they have always given me a helping hand in times of need.

A special thanks to my family. My heartfelt gratitude to my beloved husband, **Manu Singh**, for his infallible love, and constant support. Thank you for being my best friend. Words cannot express how grateful and blessed I am for my parents-in-law **Mrs. Beena Kumari** and **Mr. Virender Singh**, my parents **Mrs. Sarla Rapriya,** and **Mr. Daya Dass Rapriya** for all the sacrifices that you have made on my behalf. Your prayer for me was what sustained me thus far. I would also like to thank my siblings, **Ashish, Akanksha, Archana, Komal, and Mohit** for supporting me in everything, and especially I cannot thank you enough for encouraging me throughout this experience. To my beloved nephew, **Inu**, thank you for always cheering me up in the need of the hour.

It has been rightly said that "**Gratitude is when memory is stored in the heart and not in the mind**."

Dr. Aditi Rapriya

List of Contributors

Dr. Jitender Kumar has an experience of more than 9 years in the field of Oral and Maxillofacial Surgery. He did his M.D.S. in Oral & Maxillofacial Surgery from Pt B.D. Sharma University of Health Sciences, Rohtak. He has undergone extensive training at Regional Cancer centre, Trivandrum (Kerala) in Head and Neck Surgical Oncology. Currently working as Associate Professor in Dept. of Oral & Maxillofacial Surgery at Faculty of dental sciences, SGT University, Gurugram.

Dr. Sunil Gulia has done his BDS as well as MDS and currently pursuing his Ph.D from SGT Dental College Hospital and Research Institute, Gurugram, Haryana. He has completed Fellowship Head and Neck Surgical Oncology from AOMSI and Global Diploma in Oral Cancer from AOCMF Switzerland (IAOO). He has 36 publications in national and international journals. He has academic experience of 6 years and is currently working as an Associate Professor at SGT University, Gurugram.

Dr. Minerva Singh has done her BDS from Indira Gandhi Govt. Dental College, Jammu and went on to pursue MDS in Oral and Maxillofacial Surgery from SGT University, Gurugram where she achieved first position in University exams. Currently she is working as an Assistant Professor at her alma mater, SGT University. She has keen interest in Maxillofacial trauma, Orthognathic surgery, TMJ disorders etc.

Contents

List of Figures

List of Tables

1

Introduction

Biomimetics is defined as the study of the formation, structure, or function of biologically produced substances and materials and biological mechanisms and processes especially to synthesize similar products by artificial mechanisms which mimic natural ones.[1]

Biomimetic materials and molecules have been applied in many of the potential research areas in medical and dental sciences and highlight their foundation from plants, animals, or microbes that can be used to treat human disease.[2]

A bioactive/biomimetic material and biocompatible material is an artificial or natural material used to change part of the living system or to function in internal contact with living tissue. Bioactive materials can interact with living tissues or systems.[2]

There are several types of biomimetic materials like

Osteogenic Materials
Osteoconductive Materials
Osteoinductive Materials

Osteogenic materials include living cells that can promote the formation of new bone. Osteoconductive materials are those where the scaffold is capable of sustaining cell attachment and consequent bone matrix apposition and formation.

Osteoinductive materials are those where scaffolds support osteogenic precursor cells to distinguish into matrix bone.[2]

Osteoinduction: This term means that primitive, undifferentiated, and pluripotent cells are somehow stimulated to develop into the bone-forming cell lineage. One proposed definition is the process by which osteogenesis is inducted.

Osteoconduction: This term means that bone grows on a surface. An osteoconductive surface permits bone growth on its surface or down into pores, channels, or pipes.

Osseointegration: A process whereby clinically asymptomatic rigid fixation of alloplastic materials is achieved, and maintained, in bone during functional loading.[2]

Biomimetic Material Generations [1]

There are three different generations of biomimetic materials –

First generation of biomaterials

When synthetic materials were first used in biomedical applications, the requirements were that their physical properties should match those of the replaced tissue with a minimal toxic response of the host, so biologically inert or nearly inert materials were used to reduce the corrosion and the corrosion and the releasing ions and particles after implantation to minimize the immune response and foreign body reaction.

Examples –
Metals (stainless steel and cobalt-chrome-based alloys, Ti and Ti-based alloys).
Ceramics (alumina Al203 and Zirconia ZrO2).
Polymers (silicone rubber, acrylic resins).

The second generation of biomaterials

The second generation of biomaterials used bioactive materials 'ability to interact with the biological environment to enhance the biological response and the tissue/surface bonding', and resorbable biomaterials that cause degradation while new tissue regenerates and heals.

Example

Metals

Ceramics (bioactive glass, glass-ceramics, and calcium phosphates (CaPs)

Polymers (biodegradable polymers of synthetic and natural origin such as polyglycolide (PGA), and polylactide (PLA).

Third generation of biomaterials

The third-generation biomaterials use bioactive and bioresorbable materials as temporary three-dimensional porous structures that can activate genes that stimulate the regeneration of living tissue.

The main principle of biomimetics is to return all prepared dental tissues to full function by a hard tissue bond that allows functional stresses to allow the entire crown to its final functional biological and esthetic result.[2]

In dentistry, there is no one biomaterial that has the same, mechanical, physical, and optical properties as tooth structure and possesses the physiological characteristics of intact teeth in function. By using biomimetic therapeutic approaches, dental professionals can improve and become closer to natural biological structures and their functions.

There are two major prospective to which the term "biomimetic" is applied: a purist perspective that focuses on retreating biological tissues and a descriptive perspective that focuses on using materials that result in a mimicked biological effect. Although different, both share a common goal of mimicking biology in restoration, a biomimetic material should match the part of the tooth that it's replacing in several ways, including modulus of elasticity and function of respective area (pulp, dentin, enamel, dentino - enamel junction).

Biomaterial is any material, natural or manmade that comprises a whole or a part of a living structure or a biomedical device that performs, augments, or replaces a device that performs a function that has been lost through disease or injury. It can also be defined as any substance (other than drugs) or combination of substances, synthetic or natural in origin, which can be used for any period of time, as a whole or as a part of a system that treats, augments, or replaces any tissue, organs or function of the body. Biomaterials play an important role in craniomaxillary surgery. In order to reliably perform their desired function, biomaterial must have stable properties in a physiologic environment and must not cause adverse biologic effects on the host for reconstructive application; the selected material must possess sufficient strength to withstand cyclic masticatory and other potentially severe forces. The material and the techniques employed in their fabrication and utilization must be economically feasible. Many failures may be attributed to structural failure or corrosion of biomaterial, wound dehiscence, local tissue inflammatory reaction, or infection[3]. The functionality and compatibility of an implanted device depend on the effects of the physiologic environment on the properties of the implant and on the local and systemic histocompatibility of the implanted biomaterial. The mechanical properties of different materials may depend on stress, strain behavior, hardness, and fatigue. The chemical deterioration of the biomaterials may take place by corrosion of metals, polymer degradation, and ceramic dissolution. Tissue interaction of biomaterial would present as local (inflammation, fibrous encapsulation, infection, tumorigenesis, necrosis, and mechanical effects) and distant or systemic (migration of the biomaterial, hypersensitivity, immunologic inhibition, and accumulation of toxic element). Tissue response depends on the implant factors (composition, surface & characteristics, configuration, and mechanical aspects), host factors (species, age, site of implantation, and immunologic status), and technical factors (surgery of implantation and duration of implantation). Foreign bodies may potentiate infection by either the presence of extra inflammatory fluids and the hematomata as bacterial nutrients over those present in a normal wound or by the compromise of the tissue vascularity as a result of surgical manipulation and the pressure created by the implant or may be due to direct inhibitory or cytotoxic effects of the biomaterial on cells or humoral mechanisms mediating inflammation and healing. This book reviews the use of various biomaterials used in the field of oral and maxillofacial surgery.

2

Discussion

In the past, there was no targeted development of biomaterial based on scientific criteria. Instead devices consisting of material that had been designed, synthesized and fabricated for various industrial needs (the textile, aerospace, and defense industries) were tested in a trial and error fashion in the bodies of humans and animals. These unplanned and sporadic attempts had modest success. Most frequently, the results were unpredictable, mixed, and confounding both in success and in failure. In addition to traditional medical devices, diagnostic products, pharmaceutical preparations and healthcare disposables, now the list of biomaterial application includes smart delivery systems for drugs, tissue cultures, engineered tissues and hybrid organs. Undoubtedly biomaterial have had major impact on the practice of contemporary medicine and patient care in both saving and improving the quality of lives of the humans and animals[4].

Classification of Biomaterials[5]

Many factors are involved in the successful incorporation of a grafted material, including graft type, preparation site, vascularity, mechanical strength, and pore size of the material. The four desired properties for the biomaterial are osteogenesis, osteoinduction, osteoconduction and osteointegration.[6]

The morphology of the bone replacement grafts has been postulated to contribute to their osteoconductive capacity mainly due to influence of particle size and shape on the resorption and replacement phenomenon, as well as the influence of the interparticulate space on infiltration of vascular cellular elements and bone formation.[7]

Table 1: Characteristics of biological and synthetic materials

Biological Materials	***Synthetic Materials***
Cellular	Acellular
Hydrous	Anhydrous
Anisotropic	Isotropic
Heterogeneous	Homogeneous
Viscoelastic	Elastic
Capable of Self-repair/ Alive	Inanimate

Implant devices are placed inside the body via invasive surgical procedures that cause cell, tissue, and organ injury and thus trigger the wound healing response of surrounding vascularized tissue. Biomaterials adsorb serum-derived opsonins that mediate subsequent adhesion and activation of neutrophils and macrophages. In the attempt to phagocytize the synthetic material, monocytes and macrophages fuse and form multinucleated "foreign body giant cells". The presence and function of macrophages and/or foreign body giant cells at the implantation site during wound healing constitutes the main part of what is referred to as "foreign body reaction"; components of the granulation tissue, specifically the new capillaries and fibroblasts, are also part of this response. Fibrous encapsulation is the end stage of the wound healing process around implants.

Biomaterial surface engineering techniques are being used to modify the morphologic, physiochemical, and biological properties of biomaterials in an attempt to obtain desirable tissue-implant interactions.

Materials in Detail

Demineralized Bone

It can be used for craniofacial defects with minimal tissue reaction and remarkable little osteoclastic activity. Eight to twelve weeks after the implantation of demineralized bone, new bone growth was noticed in histologic evaluation. More bone and endothelial growth were noticed on the dural aspect of the calvaria and its continuity with the implant surface. It is believed that hydrolytic enzyme was the main causative factor of this degradation, as the fragmentation occurs in the absence of multinuclear cells. In clinical trial, demineralized bone processes with micro perforation were observed, these are believed to be centers of new bone formation, and this micro perforation may enhance osteoinduction within the implants. Several areas contiguous with non-vital bone showed evidence of transformation into living bone and remodeling. The advantages of using demineralized bone are that it is pliable, easy to shape to fit the specific craniofacial defect, and in limitless supply, and that is free from donor morbidity, which is particularly useful in pediatric patients. Properly prepared demineralized bone is a safe material for craniofacial reconstruction that eliminates the need for a second operative site to harvest a bone graft.

This material is composed of living osteoblasts derived from treated homograft materials, which theoretically provide osteogenic cells capable of inducing osteogenesis. Theoretically, demineralized bone paste can be used alone or in combination with biomaterials such as hydroxyapatite. This procedure may have advantages, as when used in combination it could provide a structural supporting matrix with cells that have osteogenic ability.[8]

Demineralised Bone Matrix (DBM)

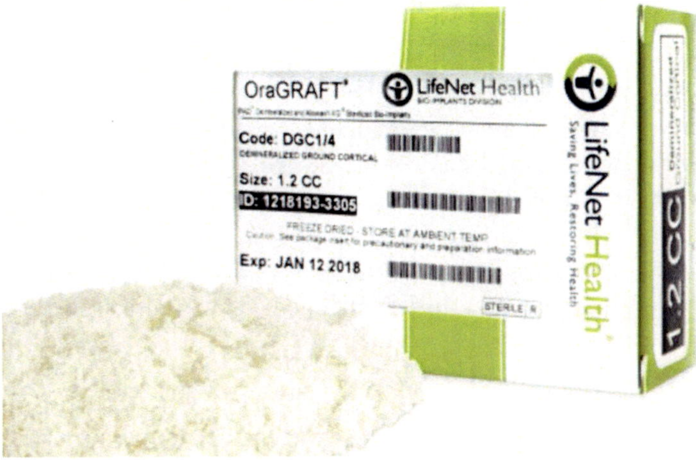

Figure 1: Demineralised Bone Matrix (DBM)

Clinically it is a good implant with inherent content bone morphogenic proteins, and is both osteoconductive and osteoinductive. It lacks antigenicity and infectivity due to the method of processing and has the ability to provide structural support and long term osteointegration of the calvaria. However, when DBM is used alone in large and subtotal cranial defects, it may require atleast one year before it becomes mineralized. Complete calvarial vault regeneration was seen only in the groups with rhBMP 2. Two factors were responsible for osteoinduction from rhBMP 2 that acted dural pericytes, inducing them into the osteogenic lineage, and osteoconduction via the DBM. Preparations such as platelet rich plasma have been reported to enhance bone grafts. These growth factors promote angiogenesis and osteogenesis, cause cells to divide, and augments production of cellular products such as extracellular matrix proteins. When combined with bone morphogenic proteins (BMP), no synergistic or additive effects were shown. Lactosorb resorbable plating is a mixture of poly lactic and glycolic acid polymerized to polymer chain with polydispersity of 2.2 and an inherent viscosity of 1.5 Dl/g. Hydrolysis of the resorbable plate progress after implantation and when the inherent viscosity reaches 0.7 Dl/g from week 6-12 and strength also decreases progressively and combine till strength is zero in about 12-15 weeks. Complete resolution in 9-15 months after surgery. Resorbable plates were used to form the struts of the geodesic framework and the inner triangular pieces were composed of pieces of DBM. This achieved both a strong framework and maximal exposure of DBM (Figure 1) to vascular tissue such as Dura and pericardium, which serve as important source of mesenchymal stem cells.[9]

Human Mineralized Particulate Bone

Particulate autogenous bone has been used to augment mandible. Control of surgically expanded soft tissue volume is believed to prevent resorption of graft material over long term. Bovine bone mixed with autogenous particulate bone combined with tissue sealant has been reported as a successful method to augment the horizontal dimension of ridge, using an open approach to place material. Human mineralized cancellous bone used for preservation of ridge width after extraction by preserving space that was previously maintained by teeth, the particular graft after 4 months has excellent ridge width sufficient to place implant.[10]

Bioactive Glass

Bioactive glass (BAG) has been used in various clinical applications. Antimicrobial BAG has the ability to attach chemically to surrounding bone; it was observed that bacteria lost their viability when placed in contact with it. It has experimentally proved property of osteoconductivity and bioactivity. BAG (Figure.2) is brittle & rigid material, it is not possible to drill, bend or shape during reconstruction operation. Preoperative mechanical preparation of brittle BAG for individual implant is difficult because of risk of microscopic fracture in BAG implant probably leading to unsafe implant.[3]

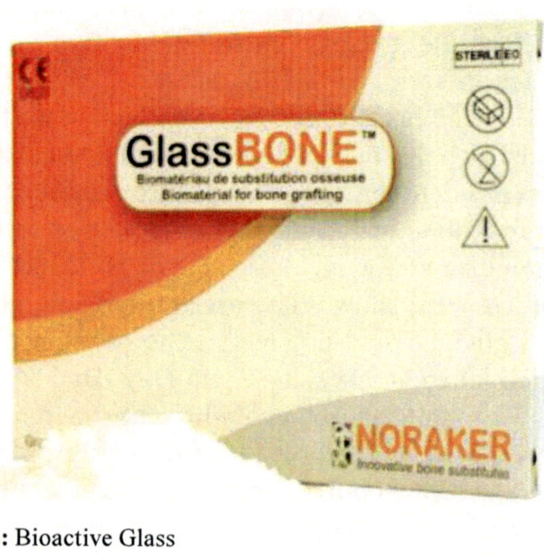

Figure 2: Bioactive Glass

Collagen Membrane

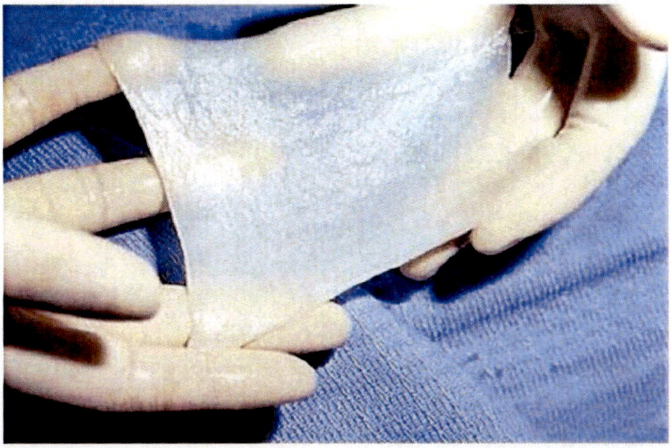

Figure 3: Collagen Membrane

Guided tissue regeneration (GTR), the procedure in which a barrier is utilized to exclude epithelium from the root surfaces, has been shown to partially regenerate lost periodontal tissue with new bone, periodontal ligament, and cementum. Several materials, both non absorbable and bio absorbable barrier, have been developed and modified, and modified in an attempt to achieve complete periodontal regeneration. More recently, the membrane barrier have also been applied for regenerating bone surrounding peri-implant defects, in the so-called guided bone regeneration procedure. Type 1 collagen is a predominant component found in periodontal connective tissue. Collagen material (Figure 3) also possesses additional advantages including hemostasis, chemotaxis for periodontal ligament (PDL) fibroblasts and gingival fibroblasts, weak immunogenicity, easy manipulation and ability to augment tissue thickness. Locci et al3 compared the degree of biocompatibility between collagen and polytetrafluoroethylene (PTFE) using H-thymidine, it was found that PTFE membrane inhibited gingival fibroblast DNA synthesis, while the matrix membrane, consisting of 95% collagen and 5 % chondroitin-4-sulfate, enhanced cell proliferation. In addition, the PTFE membrane caused a marked decrease in synthesis of extracellular collagen and glycosaminoglycan (GAG), the major component of extracellular matrix (ECM). Schiegel et al evaluated the immune responses to the collagen membrane both in vivo and in a pilot study in humans. Using enzymes-linked immunosorbent assay (ELISA), the authors found no specific immunoreaction against collagen during an 8–65 day observation period. Thus, this confirmed the lack of immunogenicity of collagen membrane previously reported by John et al0 and Wang et al. The degradation rate of collagen membranes varies depending on the source. Unsal et al compared different collagen materials including fascia lata, fascia temporalis, Dura mater, and bovine origin. The author observed that type I bovine collagen and fascia lata were resorbed faster and that the majority of material were replaced by normal connective tissue after 42 days. The resorption rates of Dura mater and fascia temporalis were much slower. To prolong the absorption time of collagen membranes various cross-linking techniques have been developed. These include ultraviolet light, hexamethylenedilsocynate (HMDIC), glutaraldehyde plus irradiation, and diphenylphosphorylazide. Collagen membrane decreases the mitotic activity of basal cells resulting in piling up of dividing cells adjacent to the membrane, thus inhibiting apical migration of the epithelium. It should be noted that once the epithelium becomes mature membrane integrity is no longer essential for tissue regeneration. Hence, the crucial period for the membrane to remain intact is during the early wound healing period when the epithelium actively migrates along root surface. When selecting an ideal material for GBR, the following requirements should be considered, wound stabilization, space creation and maintenance, protection of the underlying blood clot, and the ability to exclude unwanted tissues or cells. Lglhaut et al reported that during GTR procedures, bone and or PDL cell migration reach their peak in 2-7 days after surgery, with a decrease in mitotic activity to almost normal levels by the end of the third week. It could be implied that cells needed for regeneration arrive at the wound sites in around 3-4 weeks; therefore, the length of the time that the collagen membrane retains its integrity should be sufficient to allow selective cell repolarization. If the collagen membrane were combined with bovine HA significant bone to implant contact were seen as compared to collagen alone. Collagen sponges have also been paced beneath collagen membranes to provide space needed for new bone formation.

Dermal Graft

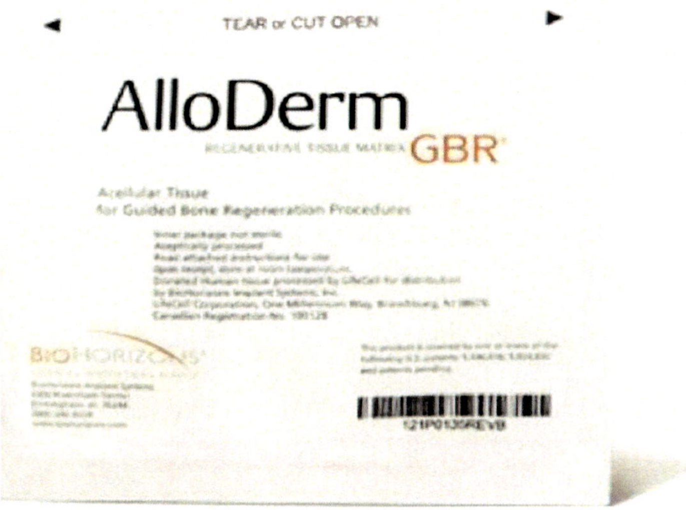

Figure 4: Dermal Graft

Neoplastic, traumatic and inflammatory diseases of the oral cavity and oropharynx frequently result in significant defects that present reconstructive challenges. Regional and distant flaps restore bulk and preserve function splint thickness skin grafts are routinely used to cover the often-significant mucosal defects arising from resection. Conventional split thickness skin grafts (STSGS) are associated with donor site morbidity, including pain, infection, and hypertrophic scar formation. In addition, full thickness defects reconstructed with STSGS are associated with significant contracture resulting from relative lack of dermis. Previous attempts at avoiding these sequelae with the use of allograft donor skin have been limited by their ultimate rejection after a short period of incorporation. Newly developed available acellular dermal matrix processed from human allograft skin. When used intraorally this processed allograft skin (Figure 4) demonstrate high % of take with host cell infiltration and neovascularization as well as epithelization from surrounding tissue. The acceptance of allograft matrix (an acellular tissue processed biomaterial acting as an immunological inert dermal transplant) is thought to result from the low immunogenicity of acellular dermal compound.[11]

Hydroxyapatite

It forms the principal mineral component of bone and constitutes 60% of the calcified human skeleton. It has been produced synthetically since 1970s and used clinically for the last 20 years. Certain marine corals have a structure that is similar to that of human bone. All forms of hydroxyapatite have excellent biocompatibility and when placed in direct contact with viable bone show osteoconduction and osteointegration. Hydroxyapatite is available in two forms; one is ceramic and the other non-ceramic[8].

Ceramic hydroxyapatite is synthesized in crystal form at low pH, and then heated (sintered) at 700 ± 1300oc to form a solid mass of X Ceramic hydroxyapatite is available in two forms; dense and porous. The dense form is entirely synthetic, it has no pores and can be fabricated into blocks or granules, which are difficult to shape and do not permit tissue ingrowth. Dense hydroxyapatite granules are difficult to contain within the desired site of implantation, and there is a possibility of migration to unwanted areas after several months or years. Porous hydroxyapatite can be produced synthetically or it can be based on the skeletons of marine corals. The calcium carbonate skeleton of the coral is chemically converted to hydroxyapatite, and the original porous structure of the coral retained. Porous ceramic granules appear to be less prone to migration over time.

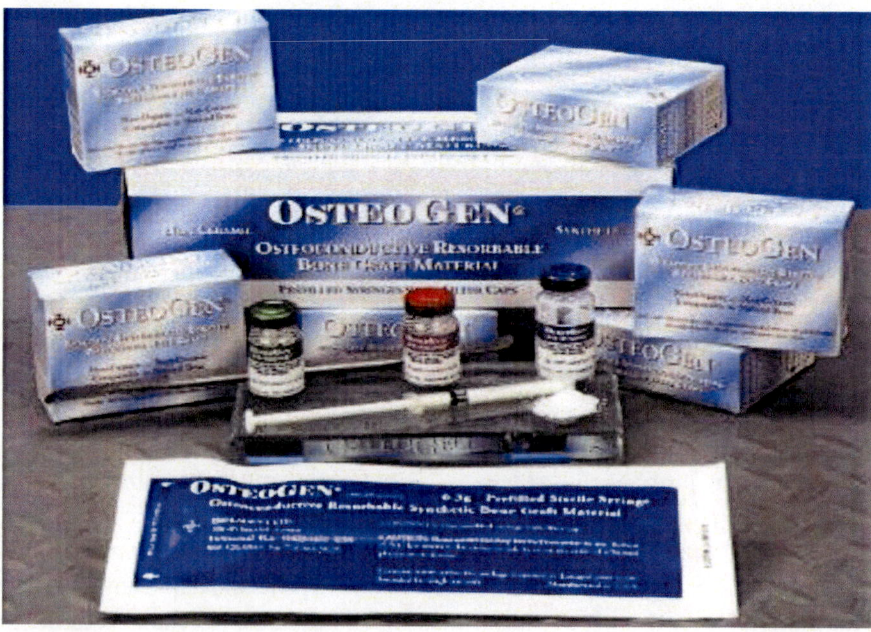

Figure 5: Ceramic hydroxyapatite

Hydroxyapatite granules (Figure 5) can be combined with Resorbable carrier compounds. The significant advantage of the porous hydroxyapatite is that it is ingrown by fibrous-osseous tissue and becomes fixed to the surrounding bone within several weeks. When fibrous ± osseous tissue ingrowth is complete, the implant consists of approximately 17% bone, 43% soft tissue and 40% of residual hydroxyapatite implant. Porous hydroxyapatite is available in block from but this is difficult to shape because it fractures easily, and it cannot be used for stress bearing application in the head and neck, so it is most appropriate as an on lay or spacer material in facial osteotomies. Because it is fragile and difficult to contour, its application has been largely limited to maxillofacial surgery, because it is fragile and difficult to contour. Porous ceramics hydroxyapatite is very versatile, in that it can be chemically combined with variable biomaterials to alter its physical properties, and it can also be used as an excellent biologically active material carrier of bioactive species, such as, bone growth proteins, which increases the ingrowth of bone into the pores[8].

Non ceramic hydroxyapatite (Tetracalcium Phosphate Cement) is the only calcium phosphate cement that sets into a stable shape and converts in vivo to pure hydroxyapatite. It is produced by direct crystallization of hydroxyapatite at physiologic pH and temperature and does not require heating to form a structurally stable implant. The dry cement is composed of tetracalcium phosphate and dicalcium phosphate, and it sets in approximately 15 minutes and converts to Ha within 4 hours. After conversion of hydroxyapatite, it is no longer water-soluble and it is slowly replaced by bone over time, without losing volume or changing shape in certain situation. Even in human trials, the cement was found to be functionally non Resorbable over 42 months on the basis of serial CT scans and by direct intraoperative inspections during secondary operations. These biologically active forms of hydroxyapatite cement are more useful in situations that are not contour sensitive or in which bone replacement of the implant is necessary, such as, in the repair of cerebrospinal fluid (CSF) leaks, translabyrinthine and trans-spheroidal defect repairs and in orthopedic applications and pediatric craniofacial surgery. Hydroxyapatite cement has disadvantages, such as a wide periosteal envelope, prolonged closed drainage of surgical fields, and granules sterile with gravity during the process, which could produce bulging under soft tissue. Injectable hydroxyapatite: after mixing hydroxyapatite granules with fibro collagen, and autogenous blood to form a paste, it can be injected into sub periosteal pocket. Although it does not osteointegration it does not become firmly fixed by fibrous tissue ingrowth. It can be used to augment malar bone, premaxillary, nasal dorsum, and glabella, and larger volumes of hydroxyapatite were used to fill craniofacial defects in children[8].

Calcium Phosphate

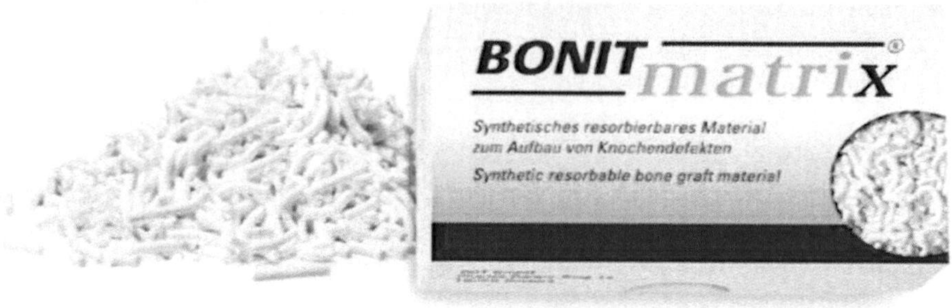

Figure 6: Calcium Phosphate

Surface reactive ceramics have been used as grafting materials and as coating in implant dentistry. Calcium phosphates in general have almost the exactly the same composition. Calcium phosphate is well tolerated, biocompatible and has osteoconductive properties. New bone formation was much stronger and faster than most bone fillers. There is bone tissue on the surface of the cement surrounding it completely, as well as within the cement. Calcium phosphate is a bioactive cement that sets as HA when moistened. Calcium phosphate cements (Figure 6) form an appetite layer on the surface shortly after implantation in the bone. The apatite particles are mixed with each other and the force linking them is weak, therefore, these particles can easily detach from the cement body, especially after dissolution has occurred. When this happens, the particles are easily ingested by osteoclast-like cells or by giant cells. Total resorption of calcium phosphate cement was seen in 16 weeks. Tricalcium phosphate are known to be usually resorbed quickly and can therefore induce an inflammatory reaction leading to scar tissue with poor bone formation. One of the main reasons for the weakness of these materials is their weakness of these materials is their porosity, which makes it easier for micro and macro cracks to run throughout the mass[13].

Calcium Sulphate

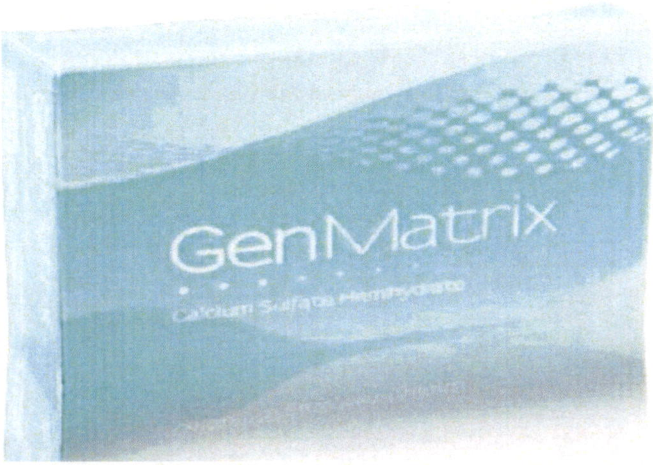

Figure 7: Calcium Sulphate

The calcium sulphate may be used as a barrier, which can halt the ingrowth of soft tissue during osteogenesis. By acting as a mechanical barrier, the calcium sulphate allowed bone cells to fill osseous defects. Bone regenerated was similar histologically and in thickness to normal bone[15]. Calcium sulfate (Figure 7) is considered as a secure material because it is absorbable, malleable, easily manipulated, and it can be used as a filler or agglutinant agent of other bone implants, in addition to presenting low cost. It can be used as a physical barrier, allowing for the osteopromotion mechanism as well as carrying out bone regeneration in controlled clinical trials and in studies with animals. One of the main advantages associated with calcium sulfate is it's in vitro biocompatibility and its tolerance to in vivo gingival tissues[14].

Fibrin Sealant

Fibrin glue was originally described in 1970 and is formed by polymerizing fibrinogen with thrombin and calcium. It was originally prepared using donor plasma; however, because of low concentration of fibrinogen in plasma, the stability and quality of fibrin glue were low. Fibrin sealant (Figure 8) can reduce bleeding and is used in almost all specialties from neurological surgery for Dural repair to vascular surgery for intraoperative control of arterial hemorrhage. Risks associated with fibrin sealants include possible transmission of blood-borne diseases. Hepatitis B and C, human immunodeficiency virus and human T-cell leukemia or lymphoma. It has been used for many years and has a wide range of clinical applications for suture support, tissue adhesion, and hemostasis. Fibrin sealant imitates the final phase of blood coagulation process. Fibrinogen is converted to fibrin on a tissue surface by the action of thrombin, which is then cross-linked by factor xiii a, creating a mechanically stable fibrin network. This fibrin network is thought to reduce the amount of postoperative bleeding by sealing capillary vessels and enabling raw operative surface to adhere. The potential advantages of the use of such substance include prevention of hematoma, reduction in surgical time, reduction in flap edema and shorter recovery time[15].

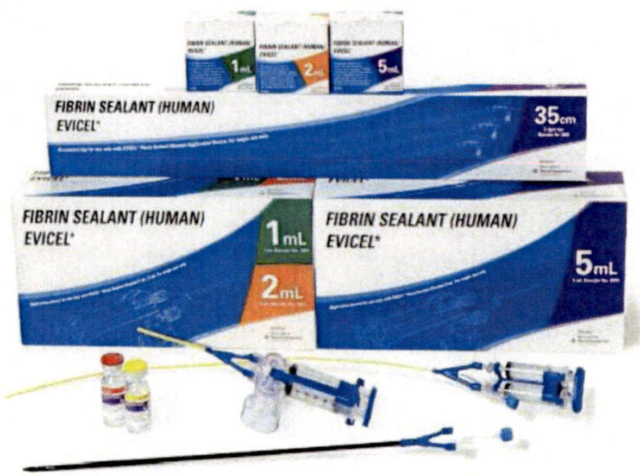

Figure 8: Fibrin Sealant

Fibrin sealant Fibrin glue as it is popularly known has been used in a number of orthopedics procedures to enhance osteogenesis in human maxillary & mandibular bone in fixation of osteochondral fractures, in spinal surgery and fixation of osteochondral fragments and bone chips. It is a derivative of blood which is widely used in surgery for their adhesive properties, hemostatic activity and wound healing process. The newly developed bone bonding agent is advantageous from the clinical application of rigid fixation technique when the use of screw is not possible. With use of adhesive fixation new trauma to delicate bone structures can be avoided during attachment to osteosynthesis plate. With new bone bonding agent and light curing bone cement the precise fixation of small and fragile fragments should be possible. The adhesive fixation technique does not lead to demineralization of bone in contrast to adhesive fixation of synthetic filling in conservative dentistry[16].

Autogenous Fat Graft

The transplantation of autogenous free fat graft into joints was reported by Murphy in 1914. He showed that autogenous free fat grafts survive and are able to protect nerves against fibrosis; he also used it in humans to prevent adhesions. According to Lexer, a fat graft shrinks in the course of 1 year, and the volume can diminish as much as two third of its original volume. It is also stated that multiple small fat grafts do not survive as well as a single large graft. There is formation of collagen fibers and hyperplasia of blood vessels taking place in fat graft which survives at the implanted site. It has been seen that the free transplants of fat implanted in spaces that would otherwise have been filled with blood or serum were not replaced by scar tissue, which will in turn into bone, but remained as soft fat tissue for months or even years. In surgery of kidney, gallbladder and liver, the free fat grafts were seen to have hemostatic properties, caused by the fast attachment of fat tissue to bleeding site, therefore stopping the bleeding. Wolford et al in 1997 presented the application of autologous fat grafting (Figure 9) in the TMJ as adjunct to prosthetic joint reconstruction in preventing fibrosis and heterotrophic bone formation[17].

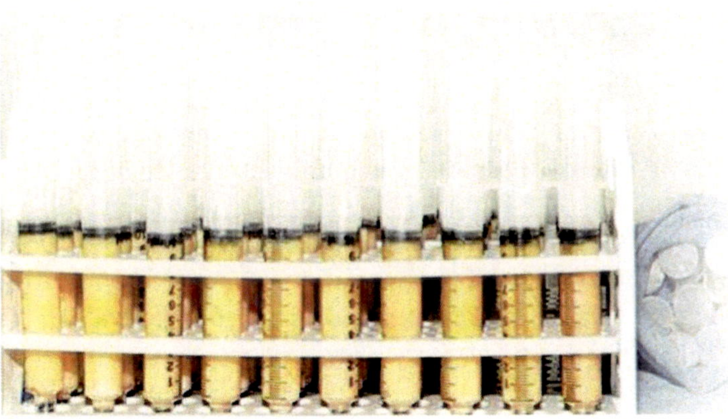

Figure 9: Autogenous Fat Graft

Polydimethylsilaxane (Silicone)

It is one of the most widely used biomaterials in the surgical field because of its soft tissue compatibility; it is easy to contour, resistant to the physiologic environment and has a wide range of mechanical properties. Surgeons can use silicone as a custom mold by mixing with hardening agent at the room temperature, the vulcanize (RTV) form of the material can be produced, either before implantation or in situ. The natural host response to the smooth surface of silicone is fibrous encapsulation, so if the soft tissue coverage is thin, unstable, or under tension the implant may be extruded. When a silicone block is used for craniofacial augmentation surgeons should be careful of silicone migration and bone erosions [8].

Polyethylene

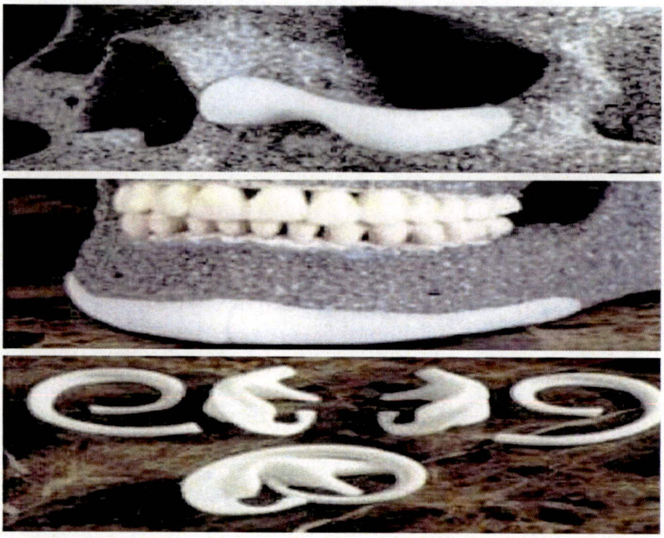

Figure 10: Polyethylene

It is available in porous form called Medpor; it has a simple linear carbon chain structure and is one of the most commonly used biomaterials over the past 25 years. It elicits a minimal tissue reaction when manufactured in its high-density with high molecular weight. The porous structure of polyethylene provides ingrowth of soft tissue after 1 week and bone after 3 weeks. Its porosity makes it easy to carve, but difficult to remove. There are many commercially available implant forms, such as, malar, chin, mandible, nasal reconstruction, and orbital implant. Flexblock, porous polyethylene is ideal suited for the repair of small to medium sized cranial defects. During operation, polyethylene implants (Figure 10) should not be placed on the fabric or come into contact with the patient's skin because the implant tends to pick up debris. Host response to polyethylene is very variable but complications are rare. Porous polyethylene has advantages over autogenous bone because it is not susceptible to subsequent change in contour secondary to bone resorption[8].

High Density Polyethlene (HDPE)

In literature it has been confirmed the use of HDPE for primary orbital reconstruction leads to low incidence of infection. He reviewed use of HDPE in defects other than those associated with acute orbital trauma. The material has also been used for secondary orbital reconstruction, temporal and cranial defects, coverage of burr holes and other remodeling defects that have occurred after craniotomies and reconstruction of the donor site deformity after the harvest of cortex calvarial bone grafts. The resultant contours are excellent, particularly when the implant is fixed with small screws. In case of temporal donor site reconstruction, they found out that there were irregularities, as well as both under augmentation and over augmentation, has been a problem. Similarly, if the skin is thin in temporal region, the edge of the implant may not only be palpable but also visible. It has been observed that there is adequate vascularity to the surrounding soft tissues, the implant will do well. In case of application in chin region, difficulty in working with this material was encountered, as there was relative lack of pliability relative to other implants such as Silastic. It does not contour to the natural shape of the bony symphysis such as that it resulted in very wide, rounded unaesthetic appearance. In case of implants in nose region, soft tissue ingrowth was promoted. It was found to be excellent alloplastic bony replacement material but should not be used under strain of functional load[12].

Methyl Methacrylate

It has been used as acceptable space filler with no resorption, and it is also stronger than the adjacent skull bone by compression and torsion testing. Methyl methacrylate has two different components, mixing powder polymer and a liquid monomer. The chemical reaction is exothermic and associated toxicity is related to the free monomer. The free monomer has direct vascular effects in experimental animals. The free methyl methacrylate monomer may also cause asthmatic reaction. When the esthetic requirement is high, methyl methacrylate delivers a predictable shape on a permanent basis without subsequent resorption. Methyl methacrylate (Figure 11) can be used in the adult with good soft tissue covering and no previous infection[8].

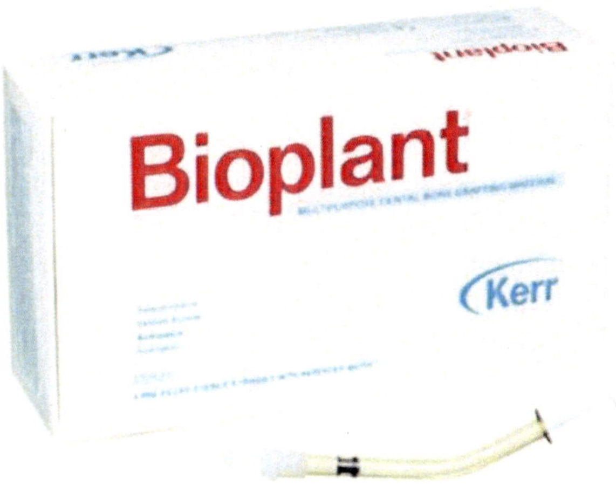

Figure 11: Methyl Methacrylate

Proplast

It is a composite material consisting of polytetrafluoroethylene combined with either carbon fibers (Proplast I) or aluminum oxide (Proplast II). As Proplast has porosity and offer the relatively inert reaction with the carbon particle, particularly when mixed with Teflon, it seems to have theoretic advantages. The clinical results with this material are not superior to hydroxyapatite, it is better than Silastic, methyl methacrylate, and other solid materials. The Proplast implant contains some growing bone, but in this situation the material was disrupted because it was not strong enough to withstand the force of the invading fibrous and osseous tissue[8].

Polytetrafluoroethylene

It has a microstructure composed of solid nodes and fibrils. Host cell migration and collagen deposition can occur between the fibrils. The current Gore-Tex product sold for facial implant is known as subcutaneous augmentation material (SAM). The advantages of Gore-Tex are that it is very pliable and evokes a minimal foreign body response with the absence of nodular scarring. Its disadvantages are that is not rigid enough to be carved. To solve these problems, the SAM implants was reinforced with layers of fluorinated ethylene propylene (FEP), which has its advantages of active collagen ingrowth, it is rigid enough to be carved, remains soft, and it is easy to remove. Gore-Tex can be used for guided tissue regeneration which is frequently used for dentoalveolar bone augmentation. The porosity of the e-PTFE provides a stable scaffold for the migration of tissue regenerating cells, which may be preferentially localized near the cranial suture lines[8].

Mettalic Rigid Internal Fixation

Metals have been used to heal wounds since dawn of medicine. In the first century, roman writer Aulus Cornelius described the approximation of a wound edge with the inserted metal pins and thread. Buck pioneered metallic fixation for the craniomaxillofacial skeleton, using intraosseous wiring to fixate a fractured mandible. Progress in the field of internal fixation, which subsided by the middle of the 19th century due to advances in germ theory, anesthesia, and antisepsis. Although the first use of rigid internal fixation with plate and screws is credited to Hansmann in 1858, the most significant advances in internal osteosynthesis were contributed by Sir William Arbuthnot Lane and Albin Lambotte Lane, a Scottish surgeon, noted early on that "no amount of traction upon the ends of the wire could retain the surfaces in accurate approximation after the grip of the lion forceps were relaxed.

Regardless of Lanes tribulations, his introduction of a "no touch" and strict aseptic technique paved the way for future of the internal fixation devices. Alloys of chromium, nickel, and molybdenum, or stainless steel and later in 1936 Vitallium paved the way due to their improved corrosion resistance. Leventhal in 1951 proposed the use of titanium for fractures. In 1967, Snell described his use of titanium hand fracture plates for the facial skeleton and Luhr introduced one of the first dedicated facial plating systems in late 1960s[6].

Stainless Steel popularized by the Champy and AO systems, comprises a mixture of iron 62.5%, chromium 17.6%, nickel 14.5%, molybdenum 2.8% and smaller amount of other metals. It is a strong and extremely rigid, making it difficult to bend and susceptible to surface damage and resultant corrosion after adaptation. After the stainless steel osteosynthesis, there is increased lymphocyte transformation, which indicates that presence of small immunologic response and the devices are biologically active in human body70. Nickel containing implants release detectable amounts of metal to the surroundings depending on factors such as type of implant, amount of metal, fracture stability, protein concentration, tissue pH, and presence of bacteria. Hypersensitivity to metal implants has been associated with ion release and accumulation of wear particles from stainless steel implants. It produced radiographic scatter more than any metal, thus was largely replaced from the mainstream of maxillofacial fixation. Today (Figure 12) it is used in form of miniplates and screws [8].

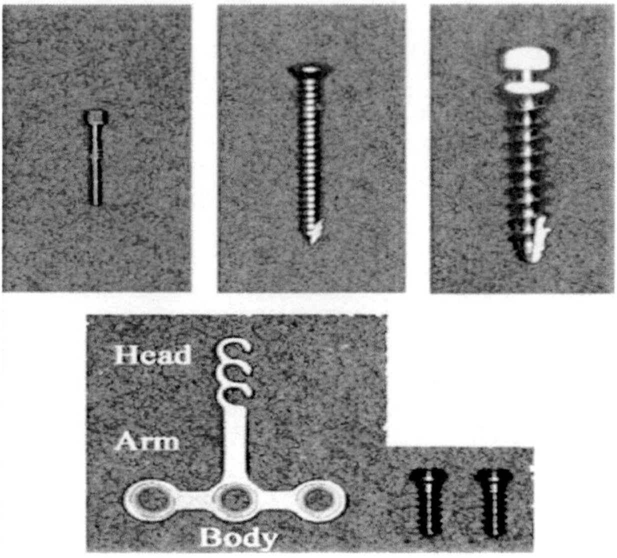

Figure 12: Stainless Steel

Vitallium is a trademarked cobalt chromium-molybdenum alloy that has twice the tensile strength, 50% more yield strength, and twice the hardness of the other metals. Plates are thinner than steel and titanium plates as on bending its yield strength doubles. It has excellent biocompatibility but produced charged inorganic compounds as corrosion products which caused tissue insult. It has limited application in orbital and maxillary reconstruction. Its popularity, however, like stainless steel, waned in spite of its strength due to difficulty adapting the thicker midface/mandible plates as a result of its rigidness and inferior radiologic scatter properties; the latter having considerable importance due to the frequent reliance on postoperative computed tomography (CT) imaging for verifying fracture reduction and plate positioning[8]. Titanium is less rigid thus is more easily adaptable, while maintaining sufficient strength. It forms an inert oxide layer around itself thus preventing corrosion and achieve good biocompatibility. It has a unique property of binding to the bone; thus, the release torque is more than insertion torque. Cost-wise, titanium hardware (Figure 13) has decreased since its introduction due to widespread use but continues to be higher than that of comparable stainless-steel components. Complications after use of titanium rigid internal fixation for craniomaxillofacial applications are most commonly associated with implant palpability, pain, or thermal sensitivity, especially when used in areas with thin skin cover. Although radiologic scatter is lower for titanium than for other metals used, titanium implants can hinder imaging or cause shielding for radiation therapy. It was seen on chemical etching and sandblasting the interfacial stiffness, removal torque and mean stiffness values increased[6].

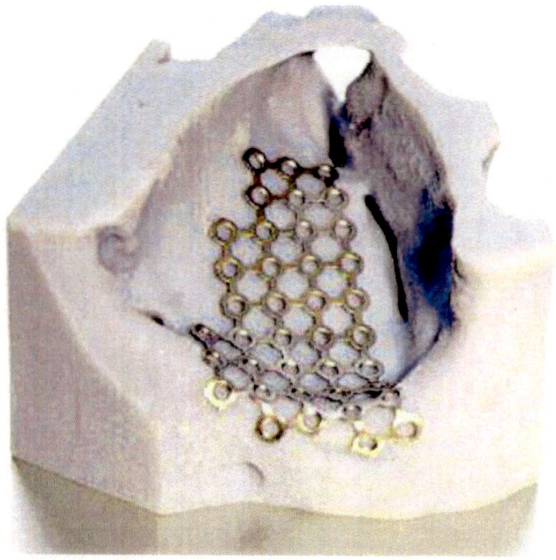

Figure 13: Vitallium

Resorbable Rigid Internal Fixation for the Treatment of Craniomaxillofacial Trauma

The development of resorbable plates and screws for rigid internal fixation was a natural extension from biodegradable suture materials already available for many years to assist wound closure. The materials currently used to manufacture resorbable plating systems in common use are polymers of high-molecular-weight a-hydroxy acids including Polyglycolic acid (PGA) and Polyglactin acid (PLA). Both materials are initially degraded by hydrolysis into lactic acid, which is then subsequently metabolized by the liver and excreted as carbon dioxide and water. However, the rate at which they degrade differs. PGA degradation is rapid and although initially stiff, loses its mechanical strength by 6 weeks and is completely resorbed within a few months. Pure PGA hardware is no longer used because its brisk structural degradation provides insufficient structural support for bone healing and is also associated with local inflammatory reaction, osteolysis, and sterile abscesses. PLA is degraded at a rate far slower than that of PGA, often requiring several years and, thus, increasing the risk of foreign body-type reactions. PLA's stereoisomers, D- and L-lactide, however, have differing degradation characteristics allowing varying combinations of these isomers to confer shorter degradation rates. In a similar manner, mixtures of PGA and PLA, with increasing amounts of the former accelerating the rate of degradation, have been formulated to achieve the same effect. From a strength perspective, the resorbable (co)- polymers with useful degradation profiles are relatively weaker and less rigid than metals such as titanium, in addition to being brittle under tensile and bending loads. To combat these structural shortcomings, resorbable plates (Figure 14) are generally broader and thicker than their metallic counterparts and often employ physical design modifications such as side rails to increase rigidity[6].

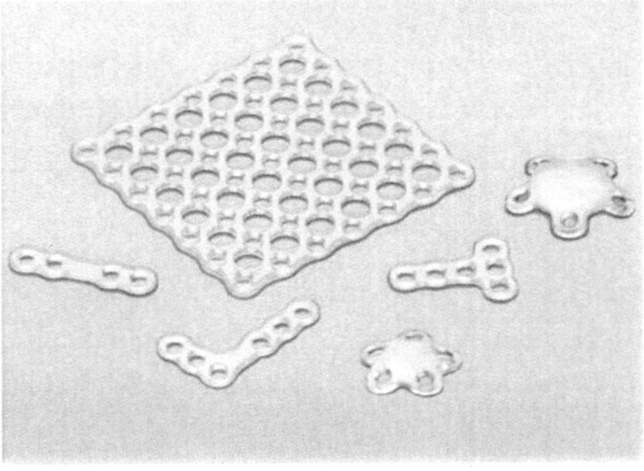

Figure 14: Resorbable Rigid Internal Fixation

Silk Fibrion

Ethiene Oliver et al assessed a new biomaterial formed from the silk fibroin protein provided biocompatibility and long-term augmentation. The material degraded slowly with negative impacts on the surrounding tissues furthermore, a biomaterial using silk fibroin protein was proven to control rate of degradation. In native fiber form, highly crystalline fibres (75% Beta – sheet content) require months to years to fully degrade because the process is a surface enzymatic hydrolysis process. Upon processing of the fibers into new material formats, the rates of the degradation were modified. Silk gels are easy to produce, biocompatibility and long lasting after implantation, represent a significant improved alternative for soft tissue augmentation. Native silk fibers exhibit tensile properties and resistance to mechanical compression that exceeds all other natural fibers and synthetic high-performance fibers. Material made of silk fibroin offer a wide flexibility in processing. Different morphologies can be formed depending on the need, such as hydrogels, porous three-dimensional matrices, nano diameter fibers and films. Hydrogels *(figure.15)* are the best type of morphology to reconstruct soft tissues, but other morphologies may be useful for other oral application[19].

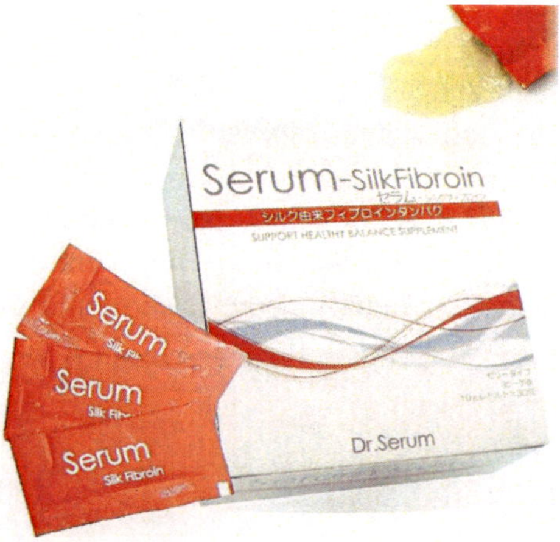

Figure 15: Silk Fibrion

Venous Blood

Peripheral venous blood was filled in view compartment under elevated sinus membrane and a spacer to induce new bone formation in maxillary sinus. Injection of Venous blood into sinus with simultaneously placed implants result in bone formation over 6 months. Histomorphometrically the amount of newly formed bone in this study was similar to higher than that achieved with bone substitutes in previous studies[20].

3

Conclusion

The craniofacial region presents a unique challenge for implantable biomaterials because the pull of the craniofacial muscles produces variable loading in different regions. In addition, craniofacial skin loses elasticity with the age and develops subcutaneous tissue sags.

Even though surgeons are familiar with the use autogenous bone grafts for craniofacial reconstruction, the usage of alloplastic bone substitutes has increased continuously, because autogenous bone is difficult to harvest, time consuming, causes significant donor morbidity, and bone resorption, but most important thing is that the biocompatibility of current alloplastic materials are improving.

Synthetic substitute creates a new avenue for clinicians to explore as adjunct in surgical procedures. These materials may not necessarily be used solely for reconstructive procedures, but when used in the right situation in combination with autologous, allograft or other synthetic, the result have the potential for more desirable results.

Unquestionably, important advances have been made in the clinical use of medical implants and other devices. Presently, emphasis is placed on the design of proactive biomaterials, that is, material elicit specific, desired, and timely responses from surrounding cells and tissues. Medical research continues to explore new scientific frontier for diagnosing, treating, curing, and preventing diseases at the molecular/genetic level. With this new fold knowledge, there will be further need for innovative formulation and/or modification of existing materials, for novel materials, and for nontraditional applications of biomaterials, such as in tissue engineering. Promising developments include bioinspired chemical and topographic modifications of materials surfaces, current-conducting polymers, and nanophase materials. In addition to new challenges and opportunities, some of the unresolved tissues of the past and present will also need to be addressed in the future.

4

Bibliography

1. Jefferies SR. 2014. Bioactive and biomimetic restorative materials: a comprehensive review. Part I. J Esthet Restor Dent. 26(1):14-26.
2. Sharma M, Murray PE, Sharma D, Parmar K, Gupta S, Goyal P. 2013. Modern approaches to use bioactive materials and molecules in medical and dental treatments. Int J Curr.Microbiol. App. Sci., 2(11):429-39.
3. Laskin Daniel M: Oral and Maxillofacial Surgery vol 1
4. Kay C. Dee, David A. Puleo, Bizios R. 2002. An Introduction to Tissue Biomaterial Interactions.
5. Peltola MJ, Vallittu PK, Vuorinen V, Aho AA, Puntala A, Aitasalo KM. 2012. Novel composite implant in craniofacial bone reconstruction. Eur Arch Otorhinolaryngol. 269(2):623-8
6. Kao ST, Scott DD. 2007. A review of bone substitutes. Oral Maxillofac Surg Clin North Am. 19(4):513-21, vi.
7. Nasr HF, Aichelmann-Reidy ME, Yukna RA. 1999. Bone and bone substitutes. Periodontol 2000. 19:74-86.
8. Rah DK. 2000. Art of replacing craniofacial bone defects. Yonsei Med J. 41(6):756-65.
9. Por YC, Barceló CR, Salyer KE, Genecov DG, Troxel K, Gendler E, Elsalanty ME, Opperman LA. 2008. Bone generation in the reconstruction of a critical size calvarial defect in an experimental model. J Craniofac Surg. Mar;19(2):383-92.
10. Block MS, Degen M. 2004. Horizontal ridge augmentation using human mineralized particulate bone: Preliminary Results. J Oral Maxillofac Surg. 62(9 Suppl 2):67-72. doi: 10.1016/j.joms.2004.05.209.
11. Herford AS, Akin L, Cicciu M, Maiorana C, Boyne PJ. 2010. Use of a porcine collagen matrix as an alternative to autogenous tissue for grafting oral soft tissue defects. J Oral Maxillofac Surg. 68(7):1463-70.
12. Semergidis TG, Migliore SA, Sotereanos GC. 1996. Alloplastic augmentation of the mandibular angle. J Oral Maxillofac Surg. 54(12):1417-23.
13. Siniković B, Kramer FJ, Swennen G, Lübbers HT, Dempf R. 2007. Reconstruction of orbital wall defects with calcium phosphate cement: clinical and histological findings in a sheep model. Int J Oral Maxillofac Surg. 36(1):54-61.
14. Silveira RL, Machado RA, Silveira CR de S, Oliveira RB. 2008. Bone repair process in calvarial defects using bioactive glass and calcium sulfate barrier. Acta Cir Bras. 23(4):322–8.
15. Mercuri LG, Ali FA, Woolson R. 2008. Outcomes of total alloplastic replacement with periarticular autogenous fat grafting for management of reankylosis of the temporomandibular joint. J Oral Maxillofac Surg. 66(9):1794-803.
16. Sanz M, Tonetti MS, Zabalegui I, Sicilia A, Blanco J, Rebelo H, Rasperini G, Merli M, Cortellini P, Suvan JE. 2004. Treatment of intrabony defects with enamel matrix proteins or barrier membranes: results from a multicenter practice-based clinical trial. J Periodontol. 75(5):726-33.

17. Rhee PH, Friedman CD, Ridge JA, Kusiak J. 1998. The use of processed allograft dermal matrix for intraoral resurfacing: an alternative to split-thickness skin grafts. Arch Otolaryngol Head Neck Surg. 124(11):1201-4.
18. Wang RC, Keech DR, Elkins TP, Russell P. 1998. The Tension Wire Method: A Simple, Effective Means of Mandibular Fixation. *Arch Otolaryngol Head Neck Surg.* 124(4):448-452.
19. Kretlow JD, Shi M, Young S, Spicer PP, Demian N, Jansen JA, Wong ME, Kasper FK, Mikos AG. 2010. Evaluation of soft tissue coverage over porous polymethylmethacrylate space maintainers within nonhealing alveolar bone defects. Tissue Eng Part C Methods. 16(6):1427-38.
20. Stadlinger B, Ferguson SJ, Eckelt U, Mai R, Lode AT, Loukota R, Schlottig F. 2012. Biomechanical evaluation of a titanium implant surface conditioned by a hydroxide ion solution. Br J Oral Maxillofac Surg. 50(1):74-9.